Health Qigong
Mawangdui Daoyin Exercises
Ma Wang Dui Dao Yin Shu

The Chinese Health Qigong Association

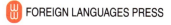

First Edition 2012

ISBN 978-7-119-07870-0
© Foreign Languages Press Co. Ltd, Beijing, China, 2012

Published by
Foreign Languages Press Co. Ltd
24 Baiwanzhuang Road, Beijing 100037, China
http: //www. flp. com. cn E-mail:flp@cipg.org.cn

Distributed by
China International Book Trading Corporation
35 Chegongzhuang Xilu, Beijing 100044, China
P.O. Box 399, Beijing, China

Printed in the People's Republic of China

Contents

Chapter I Origins and Development 1

Chapter II Characteristics 7

Chapter III Main Points 11
Section I Health-Preservation Concepts 12
Section II Hand Positions and Stances 13
Section III Breath Control and Mental Concentration 16

Chapter IV Movements 17
Section I Names of Movements 18
Section II Movements, Tips and Health Benefits 19

Initial Stance	19
Starting Stance	20
Movement 1: Drawing a Bow (*Wan Gong*)	22
Movement 2: Stretching the Back (*Yin Bei*)	28
Movement 3: Wild Duck Swimming (*Fu Yu*)	34
Movement 4: Dragon Flying (*Long Deng*)	38
Movement 5: Bird Spreading Its Wings (*Niao Shen*)	42
Movement 6: Stretching the Abdomen (*Yin Fu*)	46
Movement 7: Hawk Glaring (*Chi Shi*)	50
Movement 8: Stretching the Waist (*Yin Yao*)	54
Movement 9: Wild Goose Flying (*Yan Fei*)	60
Movement 10: Crane Dancing (*He Wu*)	65
Movement 11: Exhaling with Head Raised (*Yang Hu*)	69
Movement 12: Body Bending (*Zhe Yin*)	74
Ending Stance	80
Appendix: Acupuncture Points	84

Chapter 1
Origins and Development

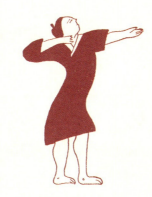

Chapter I
Origins and Development

The earliest known reference to *daoyin* exercises has been found in the *Keyi* (steeling one's will) chapter of *The Book of Zhuangzi*, a classic of the pre-Qin period (c. 2100-221 BC): "breathing in and out to get rid of the old and take in the new, imitating a bear climbing and a bird spreading its wings to prolong life – such are the practices of *daoyin* adepts and those who wish to build a better body and live as long as Peng Zu (a legendary long-lived figure)."

History also shows that practitioners who had dedicated themselves to *daoyin* and other body-building exercises were known in the pre-Qin period. According to the record, *daoyin* exercises can regulate the flow of *qi* and blood through breath control, and increase flexibility through stretching. Rich and diverse in content, ancient *daoyin* exercises can also enhance your health.

In 1973, a rectangular wooden chest was excavated from the Mawangdui Tombs (Han Dynasty 206 BC- AD 220) in Changsha, Hunan Province, containing ancient medical documents with more than 23,000 identifiable characters. During the restoration work, some broken figures were discovered, including a colored silk painting of ancient health-preservation exercises, 140 cm long and 50 cm high. The piece, drawn with figures in four rows, is about 100 cm long. There are 11 figures in each row, of an average height of 2-9 cm. Each figure shows a practitioner in realistic style, male or female, clothed or topless, outlined in black, and painted in bright red and other colors. Figures, mostly empty-handed, are accompanied by captions on their sides, 31 of which are recognizable. This painting has been identified as a map of *daoyin* health-preserving exercises and was named *Pictures of Daoyin Exercises*.

Exercises introduced in the *Pictures of Daoyin Exercises* fall roughly into five categories:

First, exercises which imitate the movements of animals, including Hawk's Glaving, Crane Crying, Dragon Flying, Macaque Calling, and Bird Spreading Its Wings.

Second, *yin* (stretching) from the word *daoyin* meant "treating disease" in ancient times. Therefore, the names of therapeutic exercises shown on the picture often start with *yin*. They serve as an aid in treating waist, knee and eye pains, abdominal ailments and deafness, and in treating pain and numbness caused by wind, cold or damp.

In the third category are exercises aiming to promote the circulation of *qi*, including exhaling with the head raised, a breathing method imitating the movement of a dragon, controlling and swallowing breath through the mouth, and a breathing method imitating the movement of a swallow.

Chapter I
Origins and Development

Fourth are exercises aiming to strengthen the body, including kicking the foot, drawing a bow, bending and stooping.

Last are massage exercises, including beating the back, a seated exercise for relieving pains of the arms and legs, and those for treating pain and numbness caused by wind, cold or damp.

Originating in a primitive society when people practiced body movements to promote the circulation of *qi* and blood and expel pathogenic cold and dampness, ancient Chinese health preservation developed from the early *daoyin* method described by Zhuangzi as "breathing in and out" and "imitating a bear climbing and a bird spreading its wings", to the forms demonstrated on the *Picture of Daoyin Exercises*. A complete set of *daoyin* exercises took shape during the Qin and Han dynasties (221 BC-AD 220), consisting of physical and breathing exercises, mental concentration and massage. Later health-preserving methods, including *Yijinjing* (literally *Book of Muscle/Tendon Change*), *Wuqinxi* (Five Animal Frolics), *Liuzijue* (a six-character formula for treating internal organ distress), and *Baduanjin* (Eight-routine Exercise), that can be traced back to the *Picture of Daoyin Exercises*, demonstrate continuity and evolution from the *Picture*.

Based on the *Picture of Daoyin Exercises*, we have selected 17 exercises. The starting stance from the *Picture* is a good preparation for the movements that follow; the final routine, i.e. folding the hands in front of the body as if holding a ball, can guide *qi* back to its origin and calm the mind. It takes about 17 minutes to practice the whole set of exercises twice. These exercises are suitable for all to practice, especially the middle-aged and the elderly.

Attached List I: Comparison of Names of Movements

Names of Movements Compared to the *Picture of Daoyin Exercises*

Movements	Names of Movements in the Original Picture	Names of Movements in this Book	Corresponding Figures
Starting Position	(Breathing Imitating the Movement of a Swallow)	Starting Stance	11th figure in the 3rd line
Movement 1	(Drawing the Hands), (Drawing a Bow)	Drawing a Bow	4th and 5th figures in the 1st line
Movement 2	(For Treating Back Pains), (For Treating Eyeball Pains)	Stretching the Back	2nd and 3rd figures in the 2nd line
Movement 3	(Wild Duck Swimming), Imitating the Movement of a Mantis	Wild Duck Swimming	7th and 8th figures in the 1st line
Movement 4	Dragon Flying	Dragon Flying	5th figure in the 3rd line
Movement 5	(Bird) Spreading Its wings	Bird Spreading Its Wings	10th figure in the 3rd line
Movement 6	(For) Relieving Discomfort of the Abdomen, (Swallow Flying)	Stretching the Abdomen	11th figure in the 1st line, 7th figure in the 2nd line
Movement 7	(Kicking the Foot)	Hawk Glaring	1st figure in the 2nd line
Movement 8	(Relieving Waist Pain)	Stretching the Waist	1st figure in the 1st line
Movement 9	(Treating Headache)	Wild Goose Flying	4th figure in the 3rd line
Movement 10	Crane (Spreading Its Wings)	Crane Dancing	3rd figure in the 3rd line
Movement 11	Exhaling with the Head Raised	Exhaling with Head Raised	1st figure in the 4th line
Movement 12	Bending Yin Diseases	Body Bending	6th figure in the 1st line
Ending Stance			

(Note: names in brackets supplied by later generations; figures numbered from left to right)

Chapter I
Origins and Development

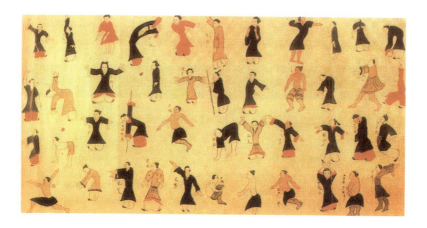

The (restored) *Picture of Daoyin Exercises* unearthed from the Mawangdui Tombs of the Han Dynasty (206 BC- AD 220)

Chapter II
Characteristics

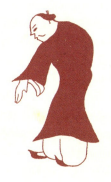

Chapter II
Characteristics

1. Focusing Attention Along the Meridians in Coordination with Mental Concentration

Ma Wang Dui Dao Yin Shu, or Mawangdui *Daoyin* Exercises have been compiled in accordance with the theory of meridians, so having a basic understanding of the meridians can help you grasp the main points of the movements while practicing. Practitioners should conduct movements while focusing their attention along the meridian pathways and controlling their breath. Mental concentration is essential while performing these movements.

2. Rotating and Stretching in a Slow, Relaxed Manner

Many movements of Mawangdui *Daoyin* Exercises aim to extend and stimulate internal organs by rotating and stretching the limbs and trunk, which benefits not only the internal organs but also the joints. Featuring slow, soft and gentle movements, this set of exercises provides easy and varied movements, most of which are rotating and stretching practices.

3. Stretching Tendons – Alternating Tension with Relaxation

By stretching the tendons and joints in a way that alternates tension and relaxation, practitioners can extend their connective tissues to the limit, making themselves more flexible.

4. Exhaling the Old and Inhaling the New – Achieving the Unity of Body and Mind

Unlike most other exercise activities, health-preserving *qigong* stresses breath control and unity of body and mind. Mawangdui *Daoyin* Exercises require practitioners to breathe naturally, concentrate the mind, and conduct movements with mental concentration to unify body and mind.

Chapter III
Main Points

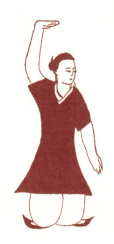

Chapter III
Main Points

Section I   Health-Preservation Concepts

1. Practicing the Exercises in an Integrated Way

Practitioners should do Mawangdui *Daoyin* exercises in an integrated way, centering on the spine to drive movements of the limbs and trunk.

2. Regulating the Flow of *Qi* Through Breath Control, Increasing Flexibility through Stretching

In order to regulate the flow of *qi* and blood, practitioners should adjust their breathing for different body movements. Breathing evenly and deeply maintains a natural and relaxed state, strengthens the diaphragm, stimulates internal organs, and improves the circulation of *qi* and blood.

In order to become more flexible, practitioners should do stretching exercises; stretching can improve flexibility and extension of all parts of the body, enhancing stability and stamina.

3. Conducting Movements Along the Meridians, Clearing the Meridians

Mawangdui *Daoyin* exercises require practitioners to conduct movements with mental concentration on meridian pathways, highlighting the role of clearing the meridians in health preservation.

Section II   Hand Positions and Stances

1. Basic Hand Positions

Palm: bend your fingers slightly, and part them slightly (Fig. 1)

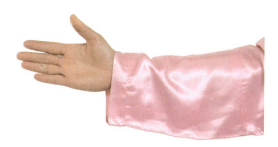

Fig. 1

Chapter III
Main Points

Hook Hand: bend your fingers naturally as shown (Figs. 2, 3)

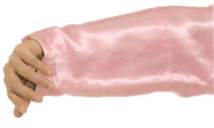

Fig. 2

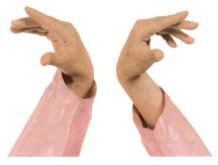

Fig. 3

2. Basic Stances

Stance with the feet horizontally apart: stand with the inside edges of your feet apart at shoulder width (Fig. 4)

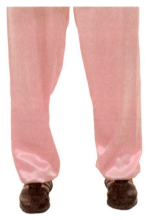

Fig. 4

Stance with a knee bent: squat with one knee bent, extend your other leg at an angle in front (Fig. 5)

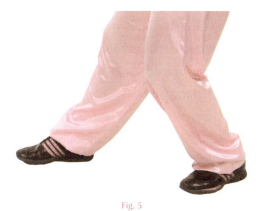

Fig. 5

Character "八 (Eight)" Stance: stand with heels touching, and extend your toes outward to form an angle of 90 degrees (Fig. 6)

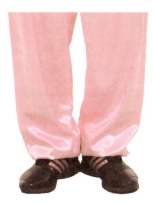

Fig. 6

Chapter III
Main Points

Section III   Breath Control and Mental Concentration

Breath control, mental concentration and the body movements are all closely linked and integrated in Mawangdui *Daoyin* exercises.

Control your breath in coordination with body movements as follows: inhale when rising or extending, exhale when lowering or withdrawing. Natural breathing (unconscious) and abdominal breathing are prescribed for different postures or strength requirements. Focus step by step to achieve the goal of even, deep breathing, and avoid excessive active control of breathing.

Mawangdui *Daoyin* exercises require mental concentration on each movement. Practitioners may adopt mental concentration step by step as they increase proficiency in the movements. Beginners should avoid excessive mental concentration, however, and regard it only as a mode of thinking while practicing health-preserving *qigong*.

For beginners of Mawangdui *Daoyin* exercises, priority should be given to body movements. The practice of mental concentration may serve as a supplemental means for novices to grasp the main points of the body movements. Practitioners may shift their attention according to different movements. For instance, when raising your hands in the starting position, keep your mind concentrated on the *Laogong* acupoints of both hands; when pressing them down, lift the *Baihui* acupoint (on top of the head) as if hanging from a rope overhead, and shift your concentration downward to *Dantian* (pubic region).

Chapter IV
Movements

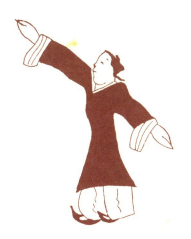

Chapter IV
Movements

Section I   Names of Movements

Initial Stance

Starting Stance

Movement 1: Drawing a Bow (*Wan Gong*)

Movement 2: Stretching the Back (*Yin Bei*)

Movement 3: Wild Duck Swimming (*Fu Yu*)

Movement 4: Dragon Flying (*Long Deng*)

Movement 5: Bird Spreading Its Wings (*Niao Shen*)

Movement 6: Stretching the Abdomen (*Yin Fu*)

Movement 7: Hawk Glaring (*Chi Shi*)

Movement 8: Stretching the Waist (*Yin Yao*)

Movement 9: Wild Goose Flying (*Yan Fei*)

Movement 10: Crane Dancing (*He Wu*)

Movement 11: Exhaling with Head Raised (*Yang Hu*)

Movement 12: Body Bending (*Zhe Yin*)

Ending Stance

Section II   Movements, Tips and Health Benefits

Initial Stance
[Movements]

Stand with your feet together, keep your head and neck erect, tuck in the chin slightly, pull in your chest and straighten your back; let your arms hang down naturally, and close your mouth, with the tip of the tongue against the palate; look straight ahead (Fig. 7).

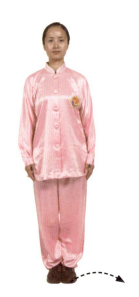

Fig. 7

[Tips]

Stand solid as a tree and breathe naturally.
Keep a calm face and a peaceful mind.

[Health Benefits]

This prepares practitioners physically and mentally for the exercises.

Chapter IV
Movements

Starting Stance

Step 1: Step your left foot half a pace to the left, placing your feet shoulder-width apart, toes pointing forward; look straight ahead (Fig. 8).

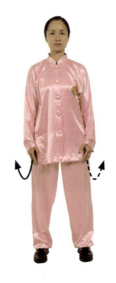

Fig. 8

Step 2: Roll your shoulders back slightly and turn your palms outward, hands facing forward (Fig. 9).

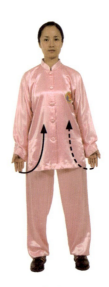

Fig. 9

Step 3: Slowly lift your hands in front of you, palms facing up, and inhale; meanwhile, raise your heels slightly, lift the hands to navel height (Figs. 10, 10c).

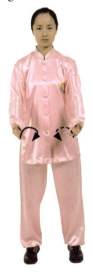

Fig. 10

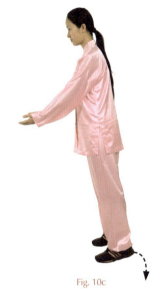

Fig. 10c

Step 4: Now slowly press your hands down to hip level, palms facing down, and exhale, letting your heels drop; meanwhile, gently press the toes into the floor (Figs. 11, 12).

Practice these hand movements three times.

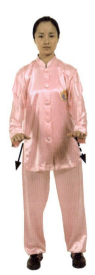

Fig. 11

Chapter IV
Movements

[Tips]

Raise the *Baihui* acupoint as if hanging by a rope from overhead, and keep your body upright and relaxed.

Change palm-down to palm-up while turning the wrists.

Concentrate the mind on *Laogong* acupoints when raising your hands, and shift your concentration downward to *Dantian* when pressing them down.

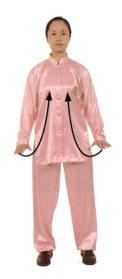

Fig. 12

[Health Benefits]

1. The hand movements accompanied by breath control can cause clean *qi* to rise and turbid *qi* to descend, and help practitioners prepare for exercise.

2. The rhythmical movements of the hands, heels and toes can improve *qi* and blood circulation, warming your toes and fingers.

Movement 1: Drawing a Bow (*Wan Gong*)

[Movements]

Step 1: Slowly lift your hands to chest height, palms up, with the fingers pointing forward and bent slightly upward; look straight ahead (Figs. 13, 13c).

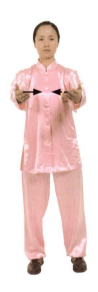
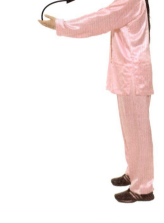

Fig. 13   Fig. 13c

Step 2: Bend the elbows to withdraw the hands toward your chest, keeping the palms at the height of the *Tanzhong* acupoint, elbows raised; with palms facing each other at a distance of about 10 cm; look forward and down (Fig. 14).

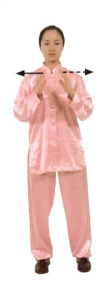

Fig. 14

Chapter IV
Movements

Step 3: Roll back your shoulders to expand the chest, and move your hands apart to shoulder width; look forward and down (Fig. 15).

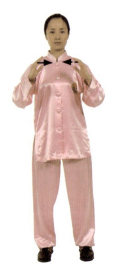

Fig. 15

Step 4: Relax your shoulders, withdraw your chest, and move your hands back to a distance of 10 cm in between; look forward and down (Fig. 16).

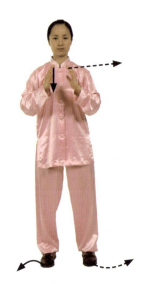

Fig. 16

Step 5: Pivot on your left heel, turning the left toes outward 90 degrees; meanwhile, turn on the ball of the right foot, turn your right heel outward about 90 degrees, and turn your body to the left. Stretch the left arm forward, palm facing up, bend your right elbow to pull the arm back as if drawing a bow, palm facing down; slightly raise your head, sway your hips to the right and let the right shoulder drop slightly; look forward and up (Fig. 17).

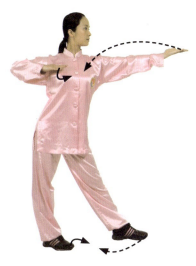

Fig. 17

Step 6: Draw the left foot back, move your right heel inward, and turn your body to the right and back to the front. Withdraw your hands to the upper chest, palms facing each other at a distance of about 10 cm in between; look forward and down (Fig. 18).

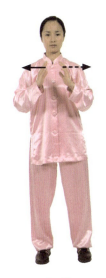

Fig. 18

Chapter IV
Movements

Steps 7-8: Repeat Steps 3-4 (Figs. 19, 20).

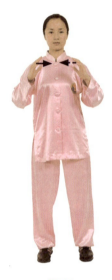

Fig. 19

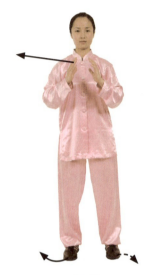

Fig. 20

Steps 9-10: Repeat Steps 5-6 in the opposite direction (Figs. 21, 22).

Do two cycles in each direction.

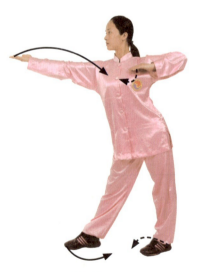

Fig. 21

[Tips]

Coordinate your movements with the breath; for example, inhale when extending and exhale when withdrawing.

Let your shoulders sag while swaying your hips; avoid too large a range of movement.

When reaching out your arm, shift your attention from the inner side of the shoulder (*Zhongfu* acupoint), via the crook of the arm (*Chize* acupoint), to the tip of your thumb (*Shaoshang* acupoint).

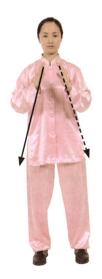

Fig. 22

[Health Benefits]

Expanding your chest, rolling back your shoulders and raising your head and hips can effectively stimulate internal organs, stretch the muscles of the neck and shoulders, and help prevent and relieve pain in your neck and shoulders.

Accompanied by breathing exercises, this exercise can help relieve chest tightness and asthma.

Chapter IV
Movements

Movement 2: Stretching the Back (*Yin Bei*)
[**Movements**]

Step 1: Let your arms hang naturally at the sides; look straight ahead (Fig. 23).

Step 2: Rotate the shoulders inward and stretch your arms forward and down to form an angle of 30 degrees with your body; then arch your back while gazing at the tips of the thumbs, and lift the heels off the ground (Figs. 24, 24c).

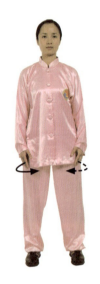

Fig. 23

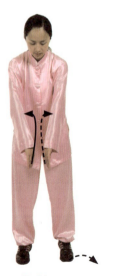

Fig. 24

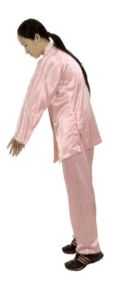

Fig. 24c

Step 3: Now drop your heels, shift your weight to the right, turn your body 45 degrees to the left and take a step forward and leftward with your left foot; meanwhile, rotate your arms outward and raise your hands to your ribcage, stroke the ribs with the backs of your hands; look forward and to the left (Fig. 25).

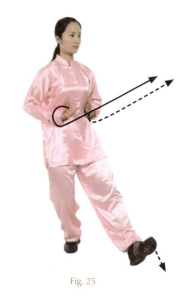

Fig. 25

Step 4: Shift your weight forward, swing your arms in an upward arc along your sides to shoulder height, with the backs of the hands facing each other to form a hook; lift the right heel off the ground, eyes looking at your hands (Fig. 26).

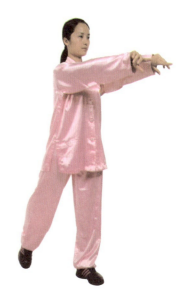

Fig. 26

Chapter IV
Movements

Step 5: Now shift your weight back, sit back on your hips, drop your right heel; slightly bend your wrists with palms facing outward, stretch your arms and hunch your back; focus your sight on the mid-point between the wrists (Figs. 27, 27c).

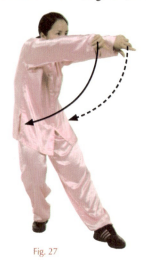
Fig. 27

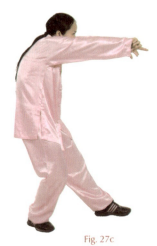
Fig. 27c

Step 6: Shift your weight forward, lift your right heel off the ground, press your hands, palms down, along the sides; raise your head and look straight ahead (Fig. 28).

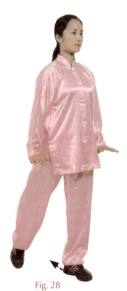
Fig. 28

Step 7: Withdraw your left foot, turn to the front, let your arms hang naturally at your sides; look straight ahead (Fig. 29).

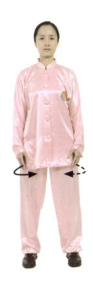

Fig. 29

Steps 8-12: Repeat Steps 2-7 in the opposite direction (Figs. 30-34). Do two cycles in each direction.

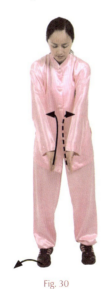

Fig. 30

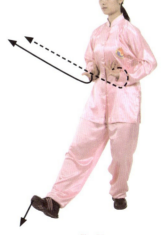

Fig. 31

Chapter IV
Movements

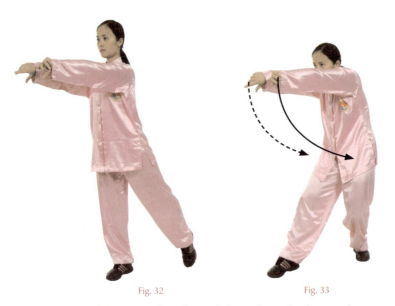

Fig. 32   Fig. 33

At the end of the second cycle, withdraw the right foot and put your feet together; look straight ahead (Fig. 35).

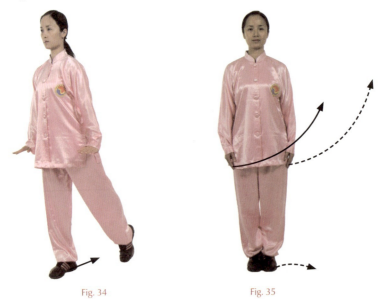

Fig. 34   Fig. 35

[Tips]

Stretch your arms and hunch your back with force, and focus on the shifting of your visual attention.

When hunching your back, shift your attention from the forefinger tip (*Shangyang* acupoint), via the outer side of the elbow (*Quchi* acupoint), to the wing of your nose (*Yingxiang* acupoint).

[Health Benefits]

1. You can fully extend your shoulder and back muscles by stretching your arms and hunching your back, which helps relax the shoulders and back.

2. Accompanied by the shifting of eyes, the practice of stretching both sides of the chest can stimulate the liver and gallbladder, and help prevent and relieve eye pain.

Chapter IV
Movements

Movement 3: Wild Duck Swimming (*Fu Yu*)

[Movements]

Step 1: Step your left foot half a pace to the left and your right foot forward to bring your feet together, and bend your knees; meanwhile, swing your arms leftward and behind your body, forming an angle of 45 degrees against the body; shift your hips to the right; look forward and to the right (Fig. 36).

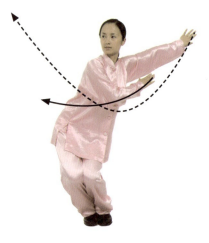

Fig. 36

Step 2: Pivot from the waist and swing your arms from left to right in an arc to your right, palm facing palm; look behind and to the right (Fig. 37).

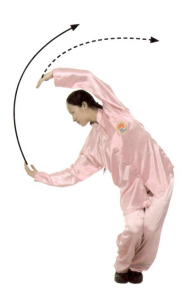

Fig. 37

Step 3: Stand upright; raise your hands above your head to form an arch, look up and forward (Fig. 38).

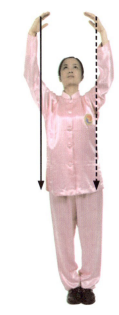

Fig. 38

Step 4: Now let your arms fall naturally along the front of the body, palms facing down, and rest them at your sides; look straight ahead (Fig. 39).

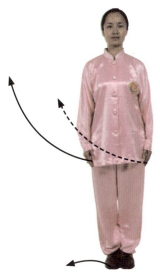

Fig. 39

Chapter IV
Movements

Steps 5-8: Repeat Steps 1-4 in the opposite direction (Figs. 40-43).

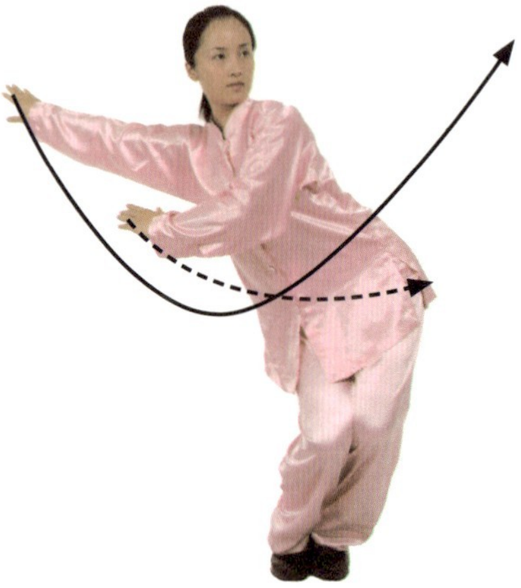

Fig. 40

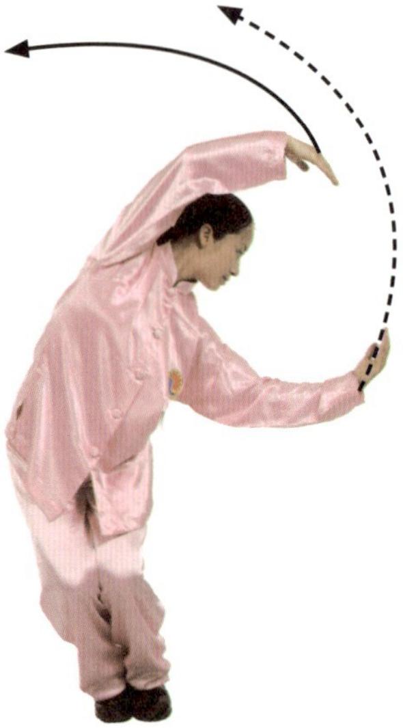

Fig. 41

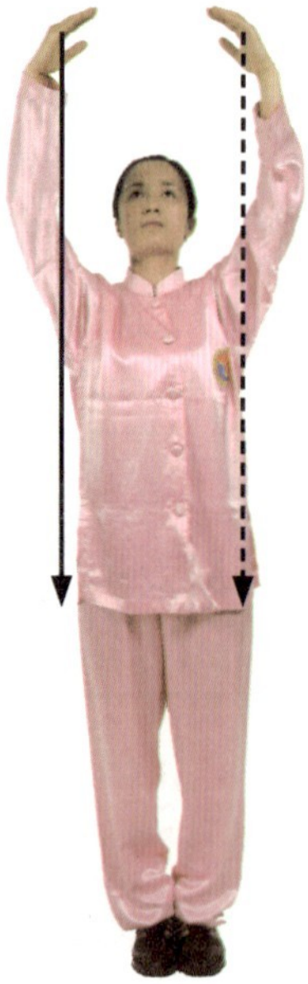

Fig. 42

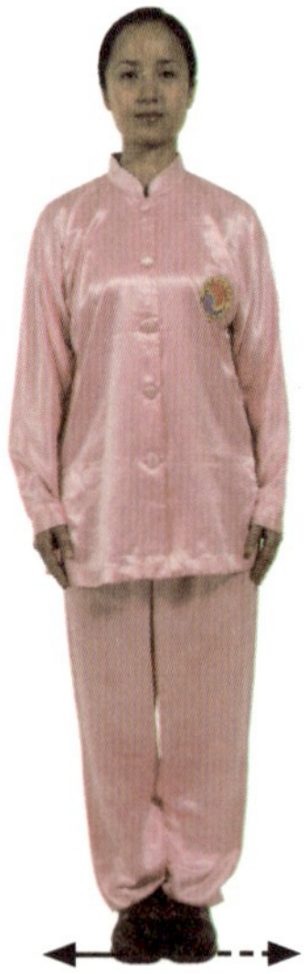

Fig. 43

Do two cycles in each direction.

[Tips]

Swing your arms within an increasing range according to your ability.

When lowering your arms, move your attention from your face (*Chengqi* acupoint) via the side of the abdomen (*Tianshu* acupoint) and the outer side of the tibia (*Zusanli* acupoint) to the tip of the big toe (*Lidui* acupoint).

[Health Benefits]

Pivoting at the waist to swing the arms and turn the body can help you lose waist fat and keep fit.

The movements of hips, arms and waist can help prevent and relieve pain in the shoulders and waist.

Chapter IV
Movements

Movement 4: Dragon Flying (*Long Deng*)
[**Movements**]

Step 1: Touch your heels together, draw the toes outward to form the Character "八(Eight)" Stance; slowly lift your hands to your sides above the waist, palms facing up, fingertips slanted upward; look straight ahead (Figs. 44, 45).

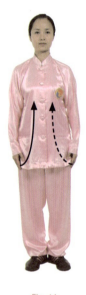
Fig. 44

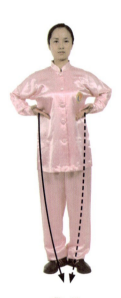
Fig. 45

Step 2: Bend your knees to squat deeply; meanwhile, push the palms forward and downward, imagine that turbid *qi* is descending; in full squat position, form the shape of a lotus flower in front of your chest with your palms facing up; focus your eyes on your palms (Figs. 46, 47).

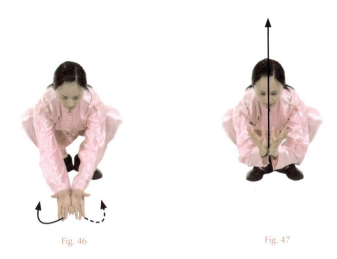

Fig. 46 Fig. 47

Step 3: Stand upright, slowly raise the "lotus" to your face, then stretch out your arms above your head; look forward and up (Figs. 48, 49).

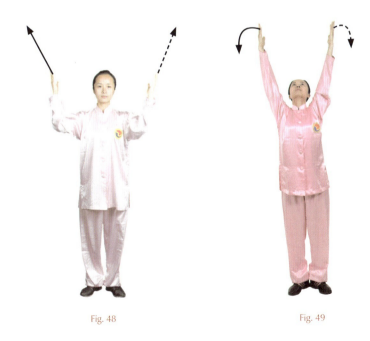

Fig. 48 Fig. 49

Chapter IV
Movements

Step 4: Turn your wrists and draw the hands outward, fingers facing outward, palms up; meanwhile, slowly lift your heels off the ground; look forward and down (Fig. 50).

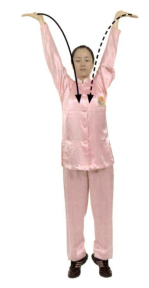

Fig. 50

Step 5: Drop your heels, press your hands, palms down, to midchest height, fingertip to fingertip, then rotate your arms outward while turning your hands over, roll back your shoulders, touch the *Dabao* acupoints with your middle fingers and look straight ahead (Figs. 51, 52).

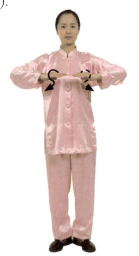

Fig. 51

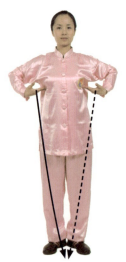

Fig. 52

Steps 6-9: Repeat Steps 2-5.

The completion of movements in squatting and standing positions is counted as one cycle; repeat it.

When finished, let your hands hang naturally at your sides; look straight ahead (Fig. 53).

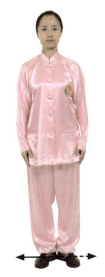

Fig. 53

[Tips]

When squatting, choose the full- or half-squat position according to your flexibility.

When raising your arms and extending your hands, lifting the heels and looking down, keep your balance and stretch as fully as possible.

When raising your hands, move your attention from the top of the big toe (*Yinbai* acupoint) via the inner side of the knee (*Yinlingquan* acupoint) to the armpit (*Dabao* acupoint).

[Health Benefits]

Arm extension can unblock the three visceral cavities, and help relieve chest tightness, obstruction of the circulation of *qi* and asthma.

Chapter IV
Movements

Heel raises in a standing position can strengthen the calf and ankle muscle groups, extend muscles and ligaments of the foot soles, and improve balance.

The stretch and squat exercise can make you more flexible, and helps relieve pain in the neck, shoulders, waist and legs.

Movement 5: Bird Spreading Its Wings (*Niao Shen*)

[Movements]

Step 1: Now, pivot on your toes, turn your heels outward, and stand with feet shoulder-width apart; rotate the arms inward, pivot at the waist to swing your arms outward, looking straight ahead (Fig. 54).

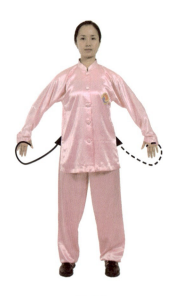

Fig. 54

Step 2: Rotate the arms outward, pivot at the waist to swing them outward within an increasing range; look straight ahead (Figs. 55, 56).

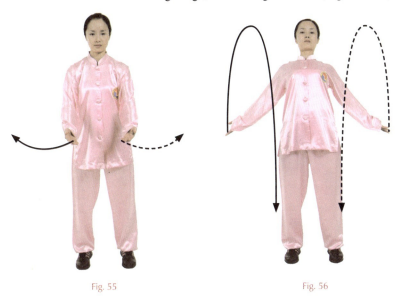

Fig. 55   Fig. 56

Step 3: Bend forward until the upper body is parallel to the ground, press the palms down in front of your body; raise your head and look straight ahead (Figs. 57, 57c).

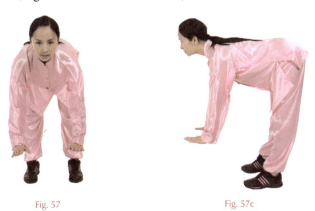

Fig. 57   Fig. 57c

Chapter IV
Movements

Step 4: Tuck in your chin, stretch the lumbar vertebrae, thoracic vertebrae and cervical vertebrae in turn; meanwhile, swing the hands forward and press them downward (Figs. 58, 58c), then raise your head and look straight ahead (Fig. 59).

Repeat Steps 1-4.

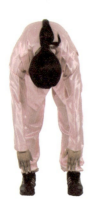

Fig. 58

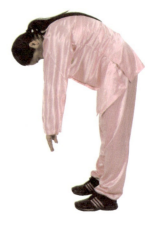

Fig. 58c

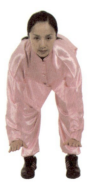

Fig. 59

Step 5: Stand upright, let the arms hang naturally at the sides; look straight ahead (Fig. 60).

Steps 1-5 count as one cycle; repeat it.

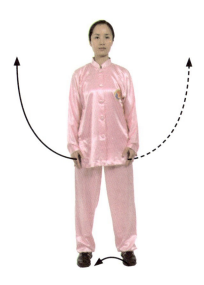

Fig. 60

[Tips]

Coordinate the movements of the head, neck and spine.

When swinging your arms, shift your attention from the armpit (*Jiquan* acupoint) via the elbow (*Shaohai* acupoint) to the tip of the little finger (*Shaochong* acupoint).

[Health Benefits]

Extending your arms forward can help prevent and relieve pain in the neck and shoulders.

Spinal exercise can help prevent and relieve pain in the waist and back.

Movement 6: Stretching the Abdomen (*Yin Fu*)

[Movements]

Step 1: Step your left foot back to put your feet together, and raise your arms, stretching them out horizontally from the shoulders; look straight ahead (Fig. 61).

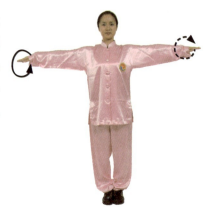

Fig. 61

Step 2: Bend the right knee slightly, sway the left hip to the left; meanwhile, rotate the left and right arms in opposite directions, turning over the palms; look straight ahead (Fig. 62).

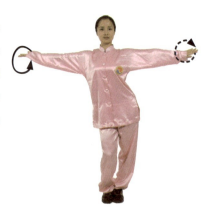

Fig. 62

Step 3: Bend the left knee slightly, sway your right hip to the right; meanwhile, rotate your arms inward and outward respectively, turning over the palms; look straight ahead (Figs. 63, 64).

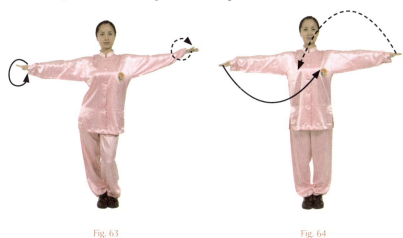

Fig. 63   Fig. 64

Steps 4-5: Repeat Steps 2-3.

Step 6: After the last exercise, move the left arm along your side in an upward curve above the head, then lower it to chest level, drop the right hand, and rotate it upward along the front of the body; cross your hands in front of your chest, left over right; look straight ahead (Fig. 65).

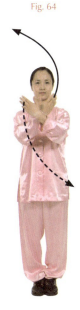

Fig. 65

Chapter IV
Movements

Step 7: Continue to rotate and raise the right hand upward until it is above your head; turn it over, fingers facing leftward, palm up, rotate your left hand outward and press it down to your left hip, palm facing down, fingers forward; meanwhile, sway your hips to the left; look forward and to the left (Fig. 66).

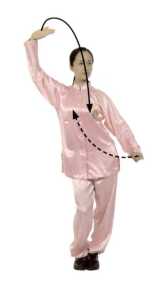

Fig. 66

Steps 8-9: Repeat Steps 6-7 in the opposite direction (Figs. 67, 68).

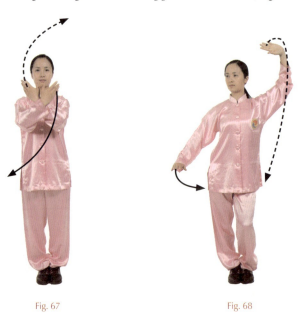

Fig. 67   Fig. 68

Step 10: Move the left palm in an outward-downward curve along the side of the body; let your arms hang naturally at your sides, put your feet together and look straight ahead (Fig. 69).

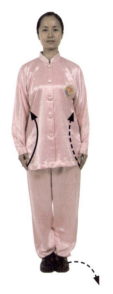

Fig. 69

[Tips]

When rotating and stretching your arms, keep your abdomen relaxed.

Lift the arms with the little finger of the upper hand pointing to the back of the shoulder (*Naoshu* acupoint) and the thumb of the lower hand pointing to your hip (*Huantiao* acupoint).

When raising your hands, shift your attention from the tip of the little finger (*Shaoze* acupoint) via the inner side of the elbow (*Xiaohai* acupoint) to the front of the ear (*Tinggong* acupoint).

Chapter IV
Movements

[**Health Benefits**]

Arm exercises can help prevent and relieve pain in your shoulders, elbows and hands.

Accompanied by arm movements, the practice of hip swaying can stimulate internal organs and help prevent and relieve indigestion and abdominal distension.

Movement 7: Hawk Glaring (*Chi Shi*)

[**Movements**]

Step 1: Turn your torso to the left, bend the right knee, and take a step forward and leftward with your left foot; rotate your hands inward to stroke the ribs (Fig. 70).

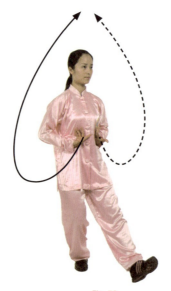

Fig. 70

Step 2: Next, raise your hands in an outward and upward arc along the sides; meanwhile, bend your left knee slightly, slowly extend your right leg forward with toes pointed outward; look straight ahead (Figs. 71, 72).

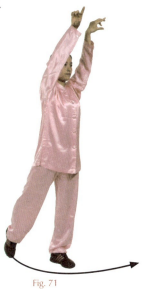

Fig. 71   Fig. 72

Step 3: Raise your arms, pull your shoulders back, crane your neck and flex your right instep to raise your toes; look straight ahead (Fig. 73).

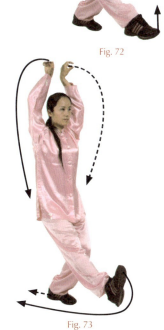

Fig. 73

Chapter IV
Movements

Step 4: Withdraw the right foot to bring your feet together; drop your arms to your sides; look straight ahead (Fig. 74).

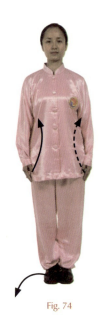

Fig. 74

Steps 5-8: Repeat Steps 1-4 in the opposite direction (Figs. 75-78).

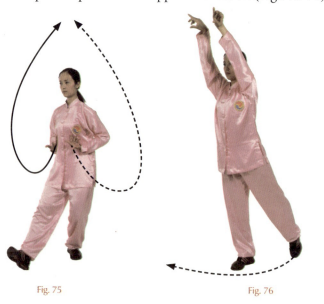

Fig. 75   Fig. 76

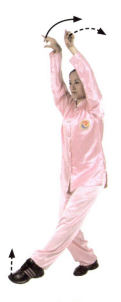

Fig. 77

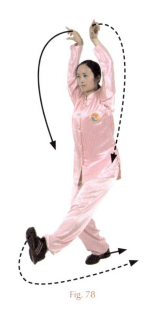

Fig. 78

Do two cycles in each direction.

At the end, withdraw your left foot, stand with feet shoulder-width apart and look straight ahead (Fig. 79).

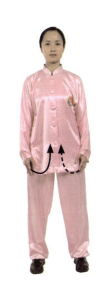

Fig. 79

Chapter IV
Movements

[Tips]

Raise your arms with palms facing outward; crane your neck slightly.

When drawing your toes back and up, shift your attention from the head via the back and popliteal space (*Weizhong* acupoint) to the tip of your big toe (*Zhiyin* acupoint); pause for a while.

[Health Benefits]

By stretching the arms, straightening the back and craning the neck you can prevent and relieve pains in the neck and shoulders.

The practice of stepping forward, and leg lifting and extension can improve your balance and help prevent and relieve leg pain.

Movement 8: Stretching the Waist (*Yin Yao*)

[Movements]

Step 1: Press your palms to the abdomen, and move them along the Belt Channel to your lower back; support the waist with your palms, push the waist forward with your fingers to arch backward; look straight ahead (Figs. 80, 81, 82, 82c).

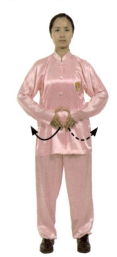

Fig. 80

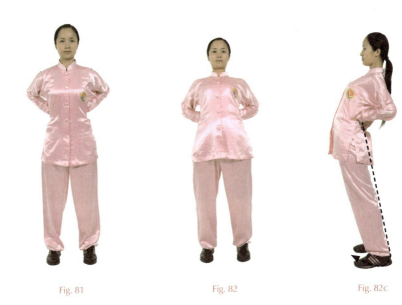

Fig. 81   Fig. 82   Fig. 82c

Step 2: Glide your palms downward from the waist to the hips; bend over, continue to glide the palms downward, via the backs of the legs, to your toes; raise your head, look forward and down (Figs. 83, 84).

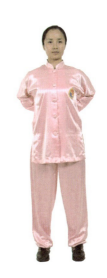

Fig. 83

Chapter IV
Movements

Step 3: Turning the waist leftward, lift the left shoulder to draw the left hand upward; meanwhile, turn your head to look to the left (Figs. 85, 85c).

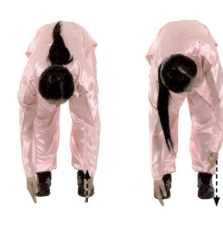
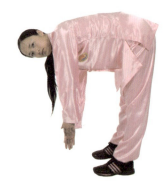

Fig. 84   Fig. 85   Fig. 85c

Step 4: While turning your waist back to the right, lower your left shoulder and hand; meanwhile, turn your head to the front, look forward and down (Fig. 86).

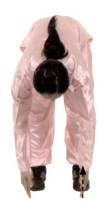

Fig. 86

Step 5: With your torso erect, rotate your hands inward, back to back, raise them along the central line to chest level; look straight ahead (Fig. 87).

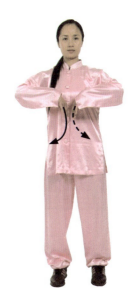

Fig. 87

Step 6: Press your palms to the abdomen, and move them separately along the Belt Channel to your lower back; support the waist with your palms, push the waist forward with your fingers to arch backward; look straight ahead (Fig. 88).

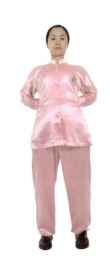

Fig. 88

Chapter IV
Movements

Steps 7-10: Repeat Steps 2-5 in the opposite direction (Figs. 89-91).

Do two cycles in each direction.

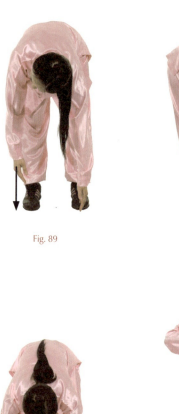

Fig. 89

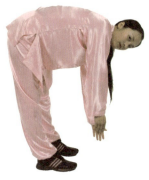

Fig. 89c

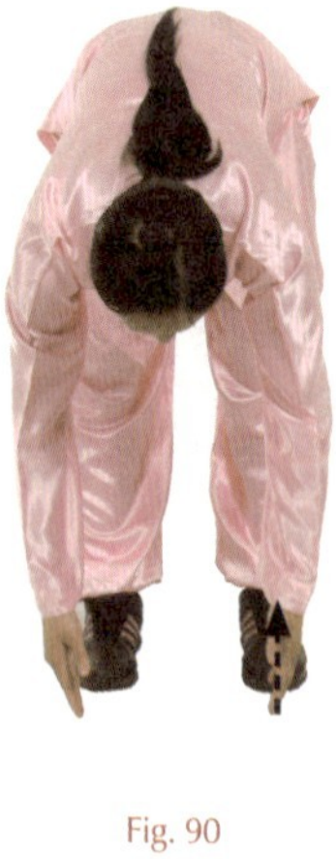

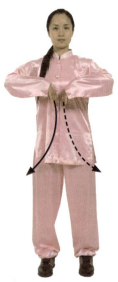

Fig. 90

Fig. 91

At the end, let your arms hang naturally at your sides; stand with feet apart and look straight ahead (Fig. 92).

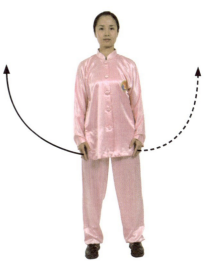

Fig. 92

[Tips]

1. Keep the right palm still when lifting the left shoulder, and turn the waist in the same direction as your head. Avoid dropping your head when bending over.

2. When raising your arms, shift the attention from the sole of the foot (*Yongquan* acupoint), via the inner side of the knee (*Yingu* acupoint), to the point beneath your clavicle (*Yufu* acupoint).

[Health Benefits]

1. The exercise of bending and turning the waist strengthens the muscles of the waist and back, and helps prevent and relieve pain in the waist and lower back.

Chapter IV
Movements

2. Accompanied by head movement, forward bending not only can strengthen the muscles of the waist and back, but also help prevent and relieve pain in the neck and back.

Movement 9: Wild Goose Flying (*Yan Fei*)

[Movements]

Step 1: Stand with your feet together and stretch your arms horizontally at shoulder level, palms facing down; eyes straight ahead (Fig. 93).

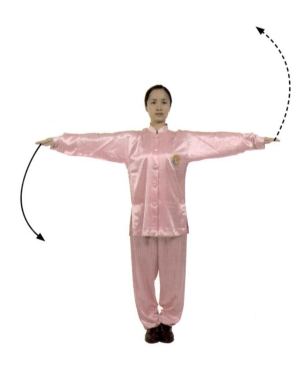

Fig. 93

Step 2: Turn the left palm up, slowly raise the left arm to form a 45-degree angle to the body; meanwhile, slowly drop your right arm; focus your eyes on your left palm (Fig. 94).

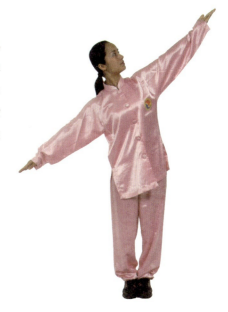

Fig. 94

Step 3: Now bend your knees and half squat, keep your arms in a straight line; and turn the head to the left, eyes looking up at the left palm (Fig. 95).

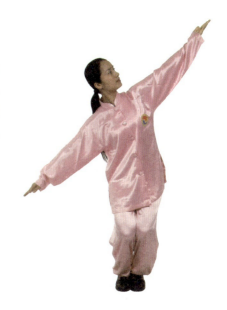

Fig. 95

Chapter IV
Movements

Step 4: Maintain this posture, turn your head to the right and focus your eyes on the right hand. (Figs. 96).

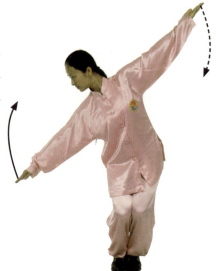

Fig. 96

Steps 5-8: Repeat Steps 1-4 in the opposite direction (Figs. 97-100).

Do two cycles in each direction.

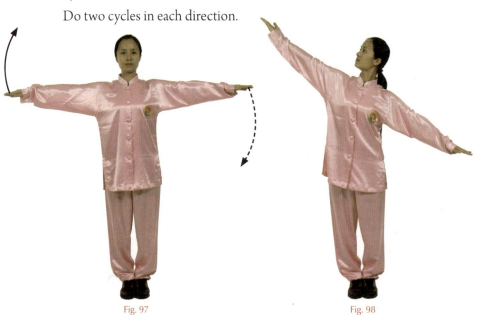

Fig. 97

Fig. 98

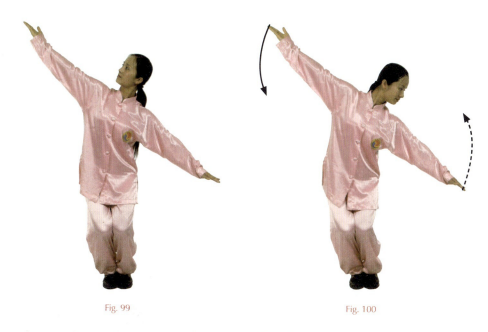

Fig. 99 Fig. 100

At the end, let your arms hang naturally at the sides; stand with your feet together and look straight ahead (Figs. 101, 102).

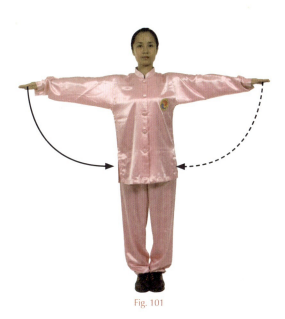

Fig. 101

Chapter IV
Movements

[Tips]

Do this exercise in a slow and relaxed way, and coordinate the movements of the hands and head.

When turning the head to look down, shift your attention from the chest (*Tianchi* acupoint), via the inner side of the elbow (*Quze* acupoint), to the tip of the right middle finger (*Zhongchong* acupoint).

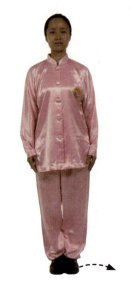

Fig. 102

[Health Benefits]

The practice of inclining to the left and right can regulate the flow of *qi* and blood, and help you relax.

Movement 10: Crane Dancing (*He Wu*)

[**Movements**]

Step 1: Bend the knees slightly with your feet apart, twist your body slightly to the right, straighten your legs, stretch the arms horizontally at shoulder height, palms relaxed and facing down; look straight ahead (Fig. 103).

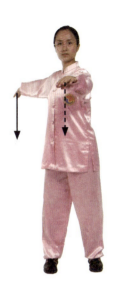

Fig. 103

Step 2: Bend your knees and half squat, slowly press your palms down; straighten your legs again and look to the right (Figs. 104, 105).

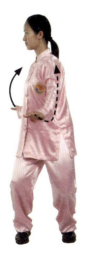

Fig. 104

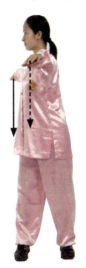

Fig. 105

Chapter IV
Movements

Step 3: Twist the body further to the right, bend your elbows to withdraw the hands, holding them upright with palms forward; bend your knees and half squat. Then slowly push the hands outward and straighten your legs again; look backward (Figs. 106, 107).

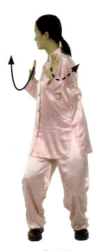

Fig. 106

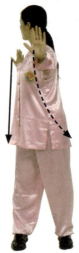

Fig. 107

Step 4: Let your arms hang naturally at your sides, turn your body to the front and bend your knees and half squat; look straight ahead (Fig. 108).

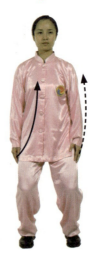

Fig. 108

Steps 5-8: Repeat Steps 1-4 in the opposite direction (Figs. 109-114).

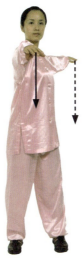

Fig. 109

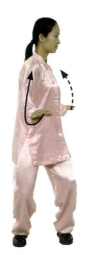

Fig. 110

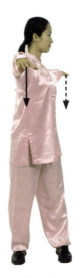

Fig. 111

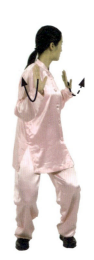

Fig. 112

Chapter IV
Movements

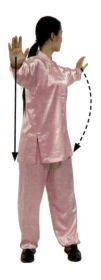
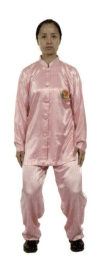

Fig. 113   Fig. 114

Do each cycle twice.

At the end, let your hands hang naturally at your sides; stand with your feet apart and look straight ahead (Fig. 115).

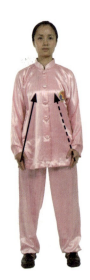

Fig. 115

[Tips]

Do this exercise in a relaxed and coordinated way.

When pushing or pressing your hands, shift your attention from the tip of the ring finger (*Guanchong* acupoint), via the outside of the elbow (*Tianjing* acupoint), to the eyebrow (*Sizhukong* acupoint).

[Health Benefits]

Arm swinging and body twisting can improve the circulation of *qi* and blood, and help prevent and relieve pain in the neck, shoulders, back and waist.

Movement 11: Exhaling with Head Raised (*Yang Hu*)

[Movements]

Step 1: Raise your arms in front to shoulder height, palms facing each other, and slowly raise them directly above your head; look up and to the front (Figs. 116, 117).

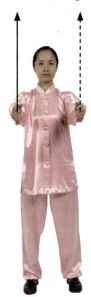

Fig. 116

Chapter IV
Movements

Step 2: Now drop your arms to horizontal, lean slightly forward, raise your head, throw your chest forward, arch your back, and look up (Fig. 118).

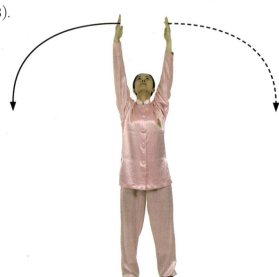

Fig. 117

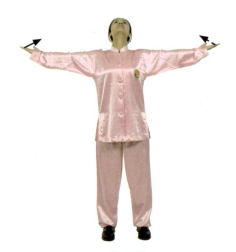

Fig. 118

Step 3: Level your head and stretch your arms outward (Figs. 119, 119c).

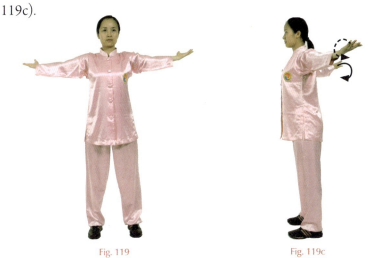

Fig. 119   Fig. 119c

Step 4: Rotate your palms while lowering your hands to your waist, fingers pointing down as you put your hands on your hips; meanwhile, slowly lift your heels off the ground, looking straight ahead (Figs. 120, 121).

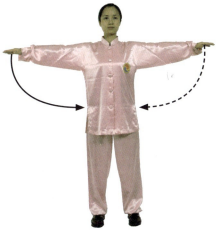

Fig. 120

Chapter IV
Movements

Step 5: Glide your hands downward over your hips while slowly dropping your heels; meanwhile, bend your knees and half squat; look forward and down (Figs. 122, 122c).

The completion of Steps 1-5 counts as one cycle; repeat it.

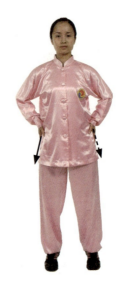

Fig. 121

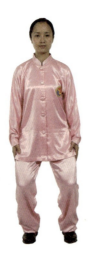

Fig. 122

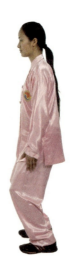

Fig. 122c

At the end, let your arms hang naturally at the sides; stand with your feet apart and look straight ahead (Fig. 123).

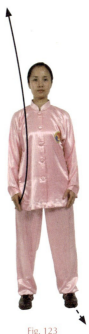

Fig. 123

[Tips]

As you lower your arms horizontally, keep your neck muscles relaxed.

When raising and lowering your arms, shift your attention from the outer corner of the eye (*Tongziliao* acupoint), via the hip joint (*Huantiao* acupoint), to the tip of the fourth toe (*Zuqiaoyin* acupoint).

[Health Benefits]

Stretching your arms backward, throwing the chest forward and exhaling can relieve asthma and chest stuffiness, and help prevent and relieve pain in the neck and shoulders.

Heel lifting can strengthen the calf muscle group, stretch the muscles and ligaments of the sole, and improve balance.

Chapter IV
Movements

Movement 12: Body Bending (*Zhe Yin*)

[Movements]

Step 1: Step the left foot forward and raise your right hand, shift your weight forward, lift the right heel off the ground and look straight ahead (Fig. 124).

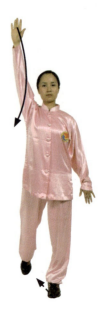

Fig. 124

Step 2: Rotate the right arm in an outward-downward curve to shoulder height, palm facing up; shift your weight backward and look straight ahead (Fig. 125).

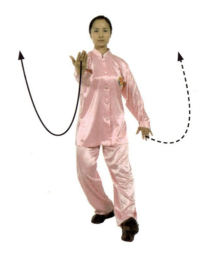

Fig. 125

Step 3: Withdraw the left foot, stretch your arms out to the sides, palms up; then turn the arms forward in front of the body, with your hands angled opposite each other at shoulder width and fingers pointing forward and inward; focus your eyes forward (Figs. 126, 127).

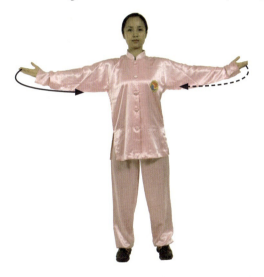
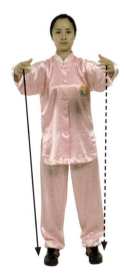

Fig. 126

Fig. 127

Step 4: Bend deeply while turning the palms downward; focus the eyes on your hands and touch your toes (Fig. 128).

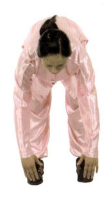

Fig. 128

75

Chapter IV
Movements

Step 5: Bend your knees, squat and lower your weight, then slowly stand up while raising your hands, palms up, to the abdomen; look straight ahead (Figs. 129, 130).

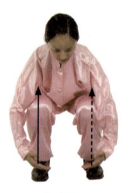

Fig. 129

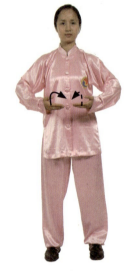

Fig. 130

Step 6: Rotate your arms inward so your palms face down; then lower your arms and let them hang naturally at your sides; look straight ahead (Figs. 131, 132).

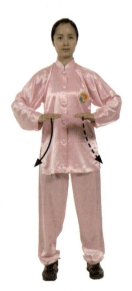

Fig. 131

Steps 7-12: Repeat Steps 1-6 in the opposite direction (Figs. 133-141).

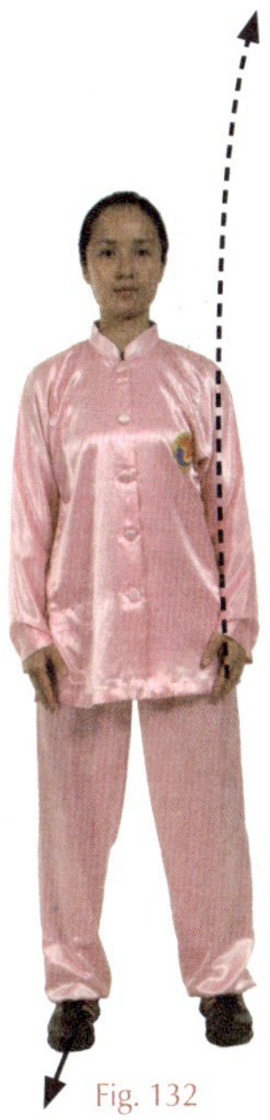

Fig. 132

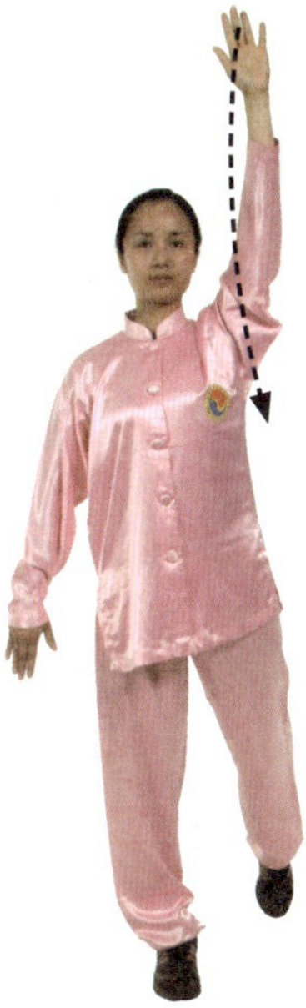

Fig. 133

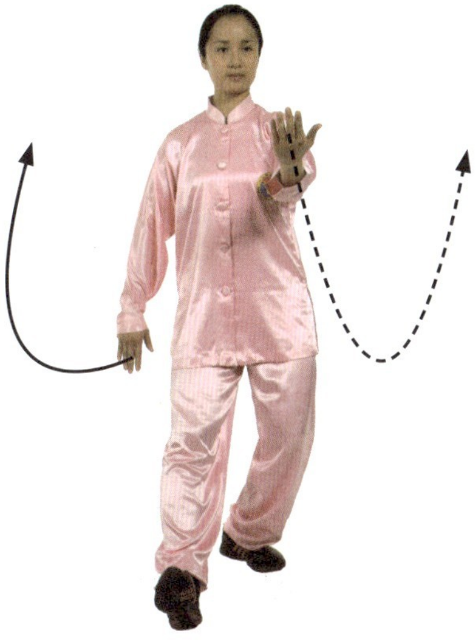

Fig. 134

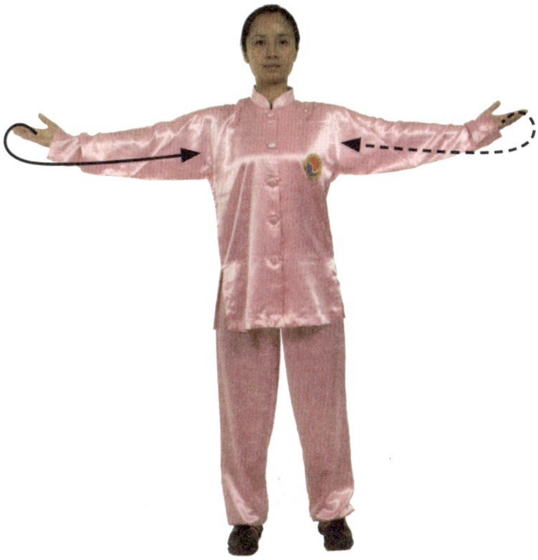

Fig. 135

Chapter IV
Movements

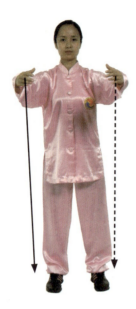

Fig. 136

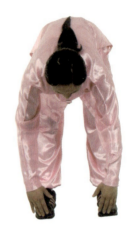

Fig. 137

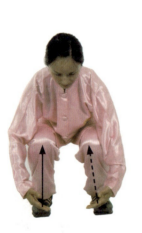

Fig. 138

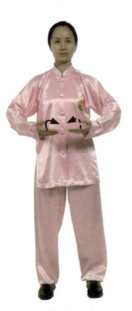

Fig. 139

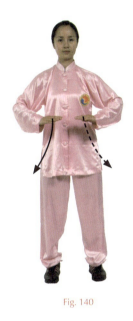 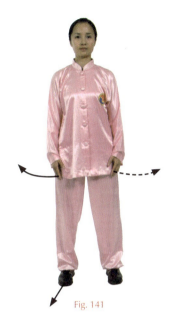

Fig. 140   Fig. 141

Do two cycles of the exercise.

[Tips]

1. When stepping forward and raising the hands, stretch the trunk as far as possible.

2. When moving your palms up along the inner legs, shift your attention from the big toe (*Dadun* acupoint), via the knee (*Ququan* acupoint), to the abdomen (*Qimen* acupoint).

[Health Benefits]

Arm stretching and dropping can help prevent and relieve shoulder pain.

Bending over can stimulate internal organs, and help prevent and relieve pain in the spine.

Chapter IV
Movements

Ending Stance

[**Steps**]

Step 1: Rotate your arms inward and swing your hands to hip height at your sides, palms facing backward; look straight ahead (Fig. 142).

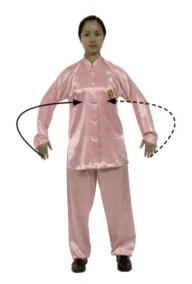

Fig. 142

Step 2: Now, raise your arms and curve them as if holding a ball, with the fingertips 10 cm apart from each other, facing each other at chest height; look straight ahead (Fig. 143).

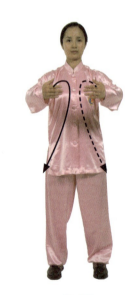

Fig. 143

Step 3: With palms facing upward, roll back your shoulders and rotate the palms inward to stroke the ribs; look straight ahead (Fig. 144).

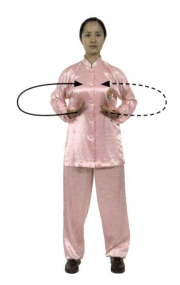

Fig. 144

Step 4: Now rotate the arms outward, fold the arms as if holding a ball with fingertips 10 cm apart from each other, facing inward at chest height; look straight ahead (Fig. 145).

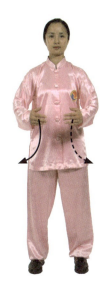

Fig. 145

Chapter IV
Movements

Step 5: Repeat Step 3.

Step 6: Now, rotate the arms outward, fold the arms as if holding a ball with fingertips 10 cm apart from each other, facing inward at navel height; look straight ahead (Fig. 146).

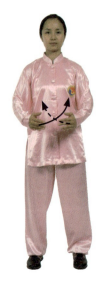

Fig. 146

Step 7: Cross your hands and overlap them at the thumbs, left over right, press them against the navel; look straight ahead (Fig. 147).

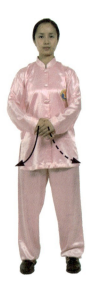

Fig. 147

Step 8: Separate your hands, press them along the Belt Channel to the hips and let them hang naturally at your sides; put your feet together; look straight ahead (Figs. 148, 149).

[Tips]

When folding your arms in front of you, shift your weight slightly forward.

Let your palms face the chest (*Tanzhong* acupoint), upper abdomen (*Zhongwan* acupoint), and lower abdomen (*Shenque* acupoint) in turn.

When pressing down your hands, focus your attention on *Yongquan* acupoint (on the sole of the foot).

[Health Benefits]

Focusing attention on *Yongquan* acupoint can regulate the flow of *qi*.

Guiding *qi* back to its origin can help you attain mental tranquility.

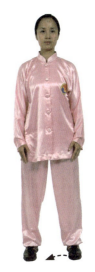

Fig. 148

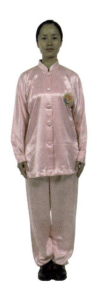

Fig. 149

Appendix
Acupuncture Points

APPENDIX
ACUPUNCTURE POINTS

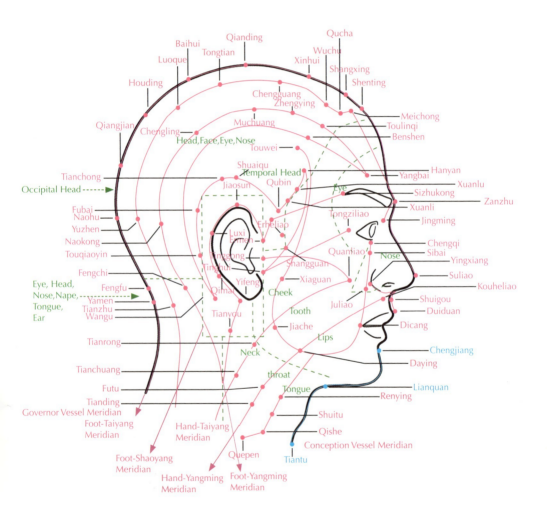

Acupoints on the head and face

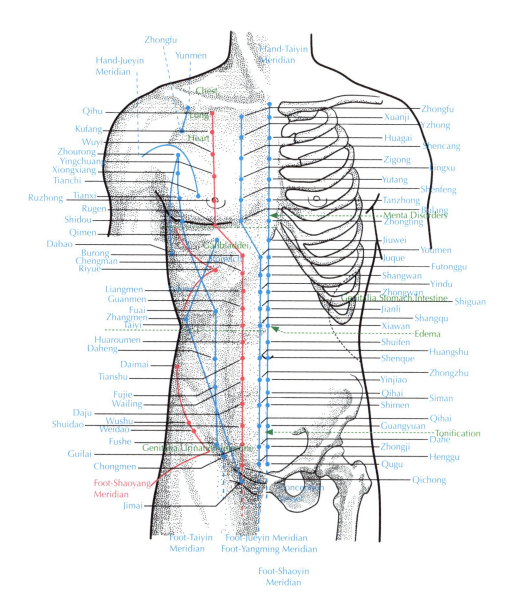

Acupoints at the chest and abdomen

Appendix
Acupuncture Points

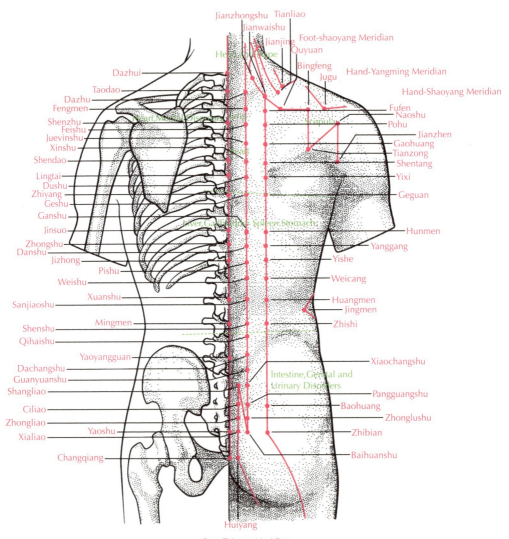

Acupoints on the back and at lumber region

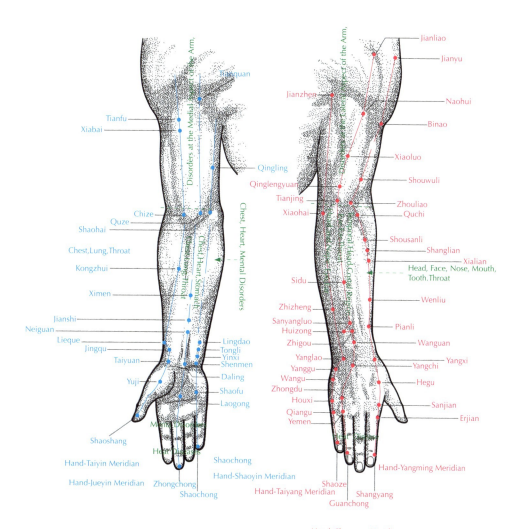

Acupoints in the upper limbs

Appendix
Acupuncture Points

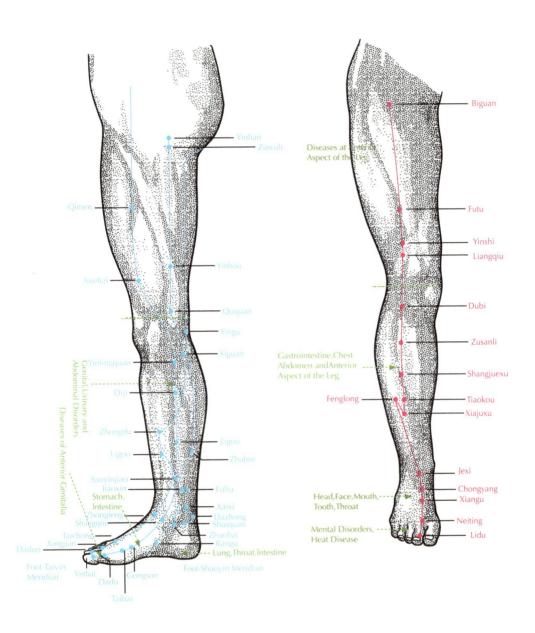

Acupoints in the lower limbs

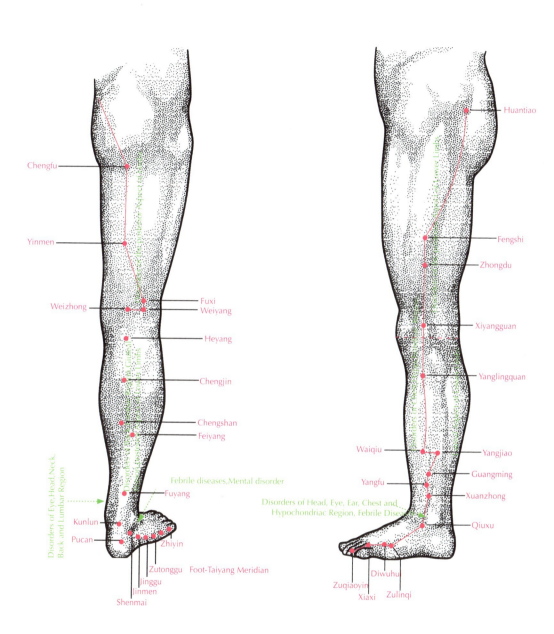

Acupoints in the lower limbs

图书在版编目（CIP）数据

健身气功. 马王堆导引术：英文 / 国家体育总局健身气功管理中心编著.
-- 北京：外文出版社, 2012
ISBN 978-7-119-07870-0

Ⅰ.①健… Ⅱ.①国… Ⅲ.①气功—健身运动—英文
②导引—英文 Ⅳ.①R214

中国版本图书馆CIP数据核字(2012)第156117号

英文翻译：严　晶
英文审定：John Stafford　　David Ferguson　　徐明强
责任编辑：杨春燕　杨　璐
装帧设计：吾昱设计工作室
印刷监制：张国祥

健身气功——马王堆导引术

国家体育总局健身气功管理中心　编

©2012外文出版社有限责任公司
出 版 人：徐　步
出版发行：
外文出版社有限责任公司（中国北京百万庄大街24号 100037）

网　　址：http://www.flp.com.cn
电　　话：008610－68320579（总编室）
　　　　　008610－68995852（发行部）
　　　　　008610－68327750（版权部）
印　　刷：北京雷杰印刷有限公司
开　　本：787mm×1092mm　1/16　　印张：6
2012年7月第1版 第1次印刷
（英）
ISBN 978-7-119-07870-0
08500（平）

版权所有　侵权必究　有印装问题可随时调换